# Mia's Mountain Hike

## A Forest Yoga Book for Kids

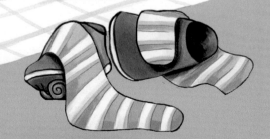

Written by Giselle Shardlow
Illustrated by Lauren Hughes

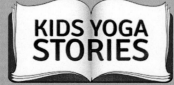

KIDS YOGA
STORIES

www.kidsyogastories.com

For my husband, my mountain hiking partner.

~ G.S.

ISBN-13: 978-1532852923
ISBN-10: 1532852924

Kids Yoga Stories
Boston, MA
www.kidsyogastories.com
www.amazon.com/author/giselleshardlow
Email us at info@kidsyogastories.com.

Ordering Information: Special discounts are available on quantity purchases by contacting the publisher at the email address above.

What do you think? Let us know what you think of *Mia's Mountain Hike* at feedback@kidsyogastories.com.

Printed in the United States of America.

# How to Use this Yoga Book for Kids

Welcome to Kids Yoga Stories. Our yoga books are designed to integrate learning, movement, and fun. Below are a few tips for getting the most out of this forest yoga book:

1. *Flip* through the story to familiarize yourself with the format. Pay special attention to the yoga pose in the circle on each page. Each pose has a corresponding keyword.

2. *Read* the story with your child, but this time, act out the story as you go along. Use the illustrations of Mia doing the poses as a guide. Encourage your child's imagination.

3. *Refer* to the list of yoga poses for kids and the parent-teacher guide at the back of the book for further information.

Enjoy your yoga story, but please be safe!

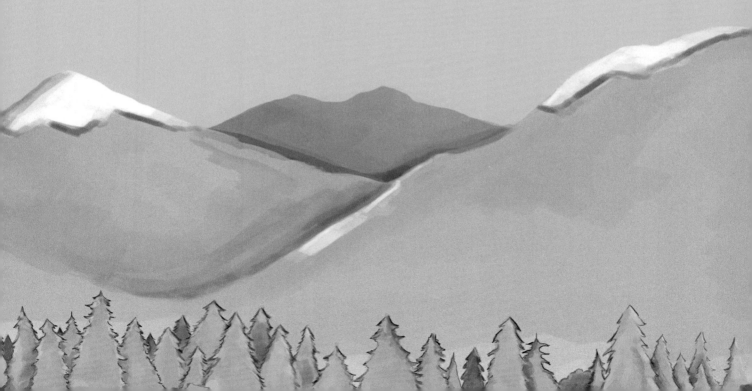

Mia loved the forest.

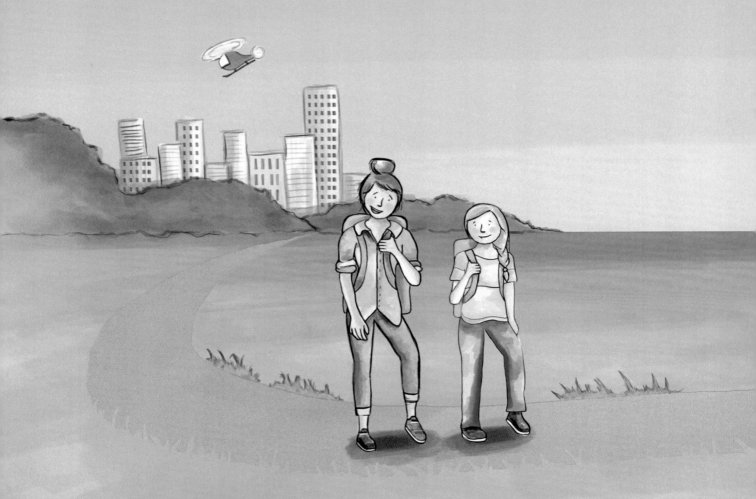

She loved looking for animals,
swimming in the lake,
and having lunch outside.

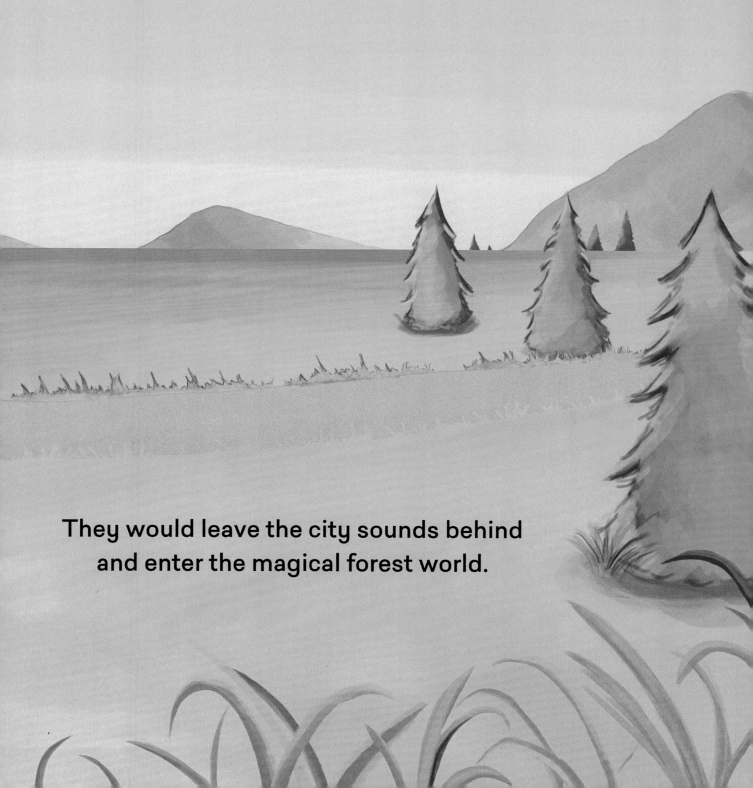

But her absolute favorite thing to do
in the forest was to go hiking with Auntie Lisa.

They would leave the city sounds behind
and enter the magical forest world.

At the head of the trail,
Mia grabbed Auntie Lisa's hand.

She smiled and then led her aunt down the mountain path.

They were off on their next adventure!

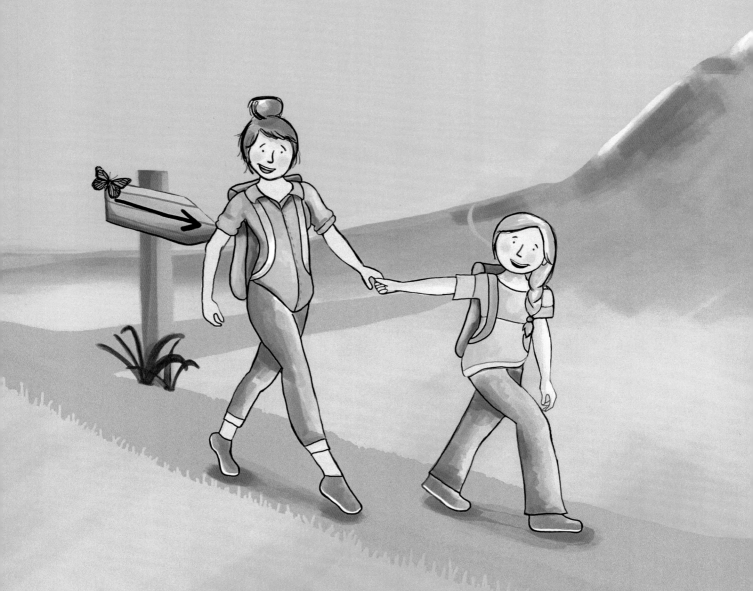

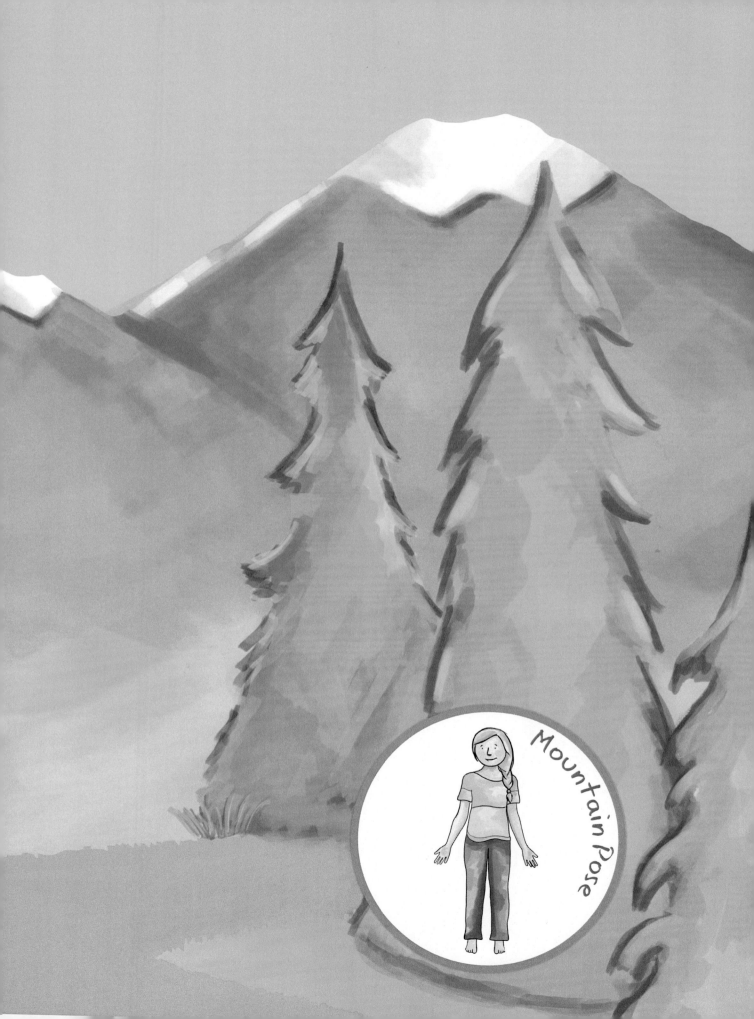

Mountain Pose

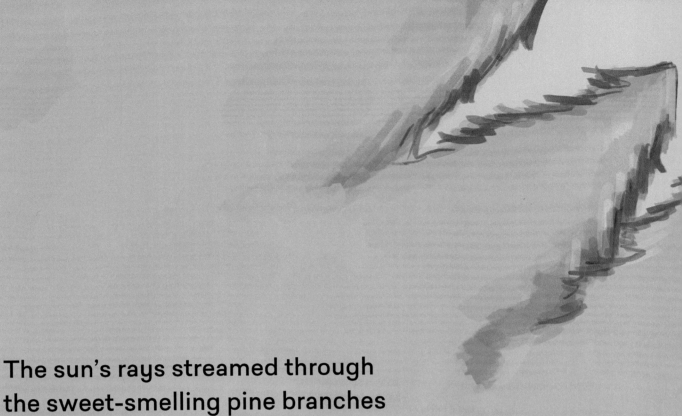

The sun's rays streamed through the sweet-smelling pine branches and lit the path.

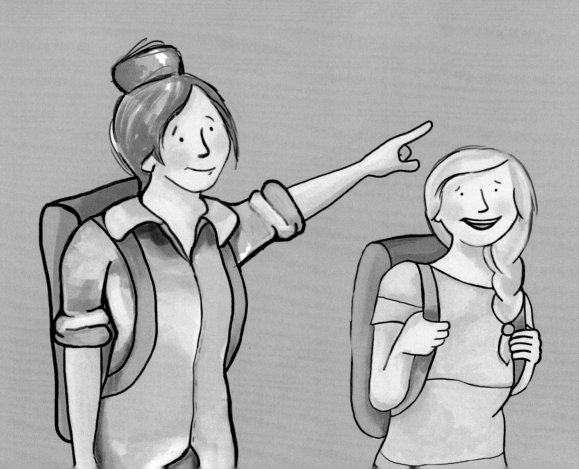

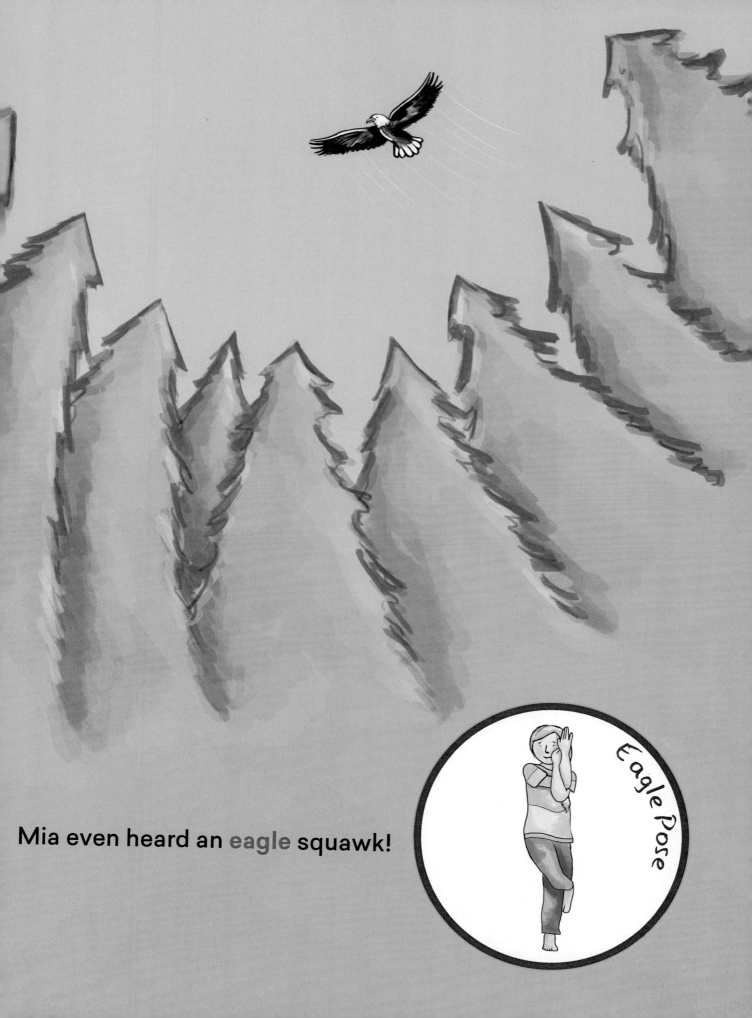

Mia even heard an eagle squawk!

Eagle Pose

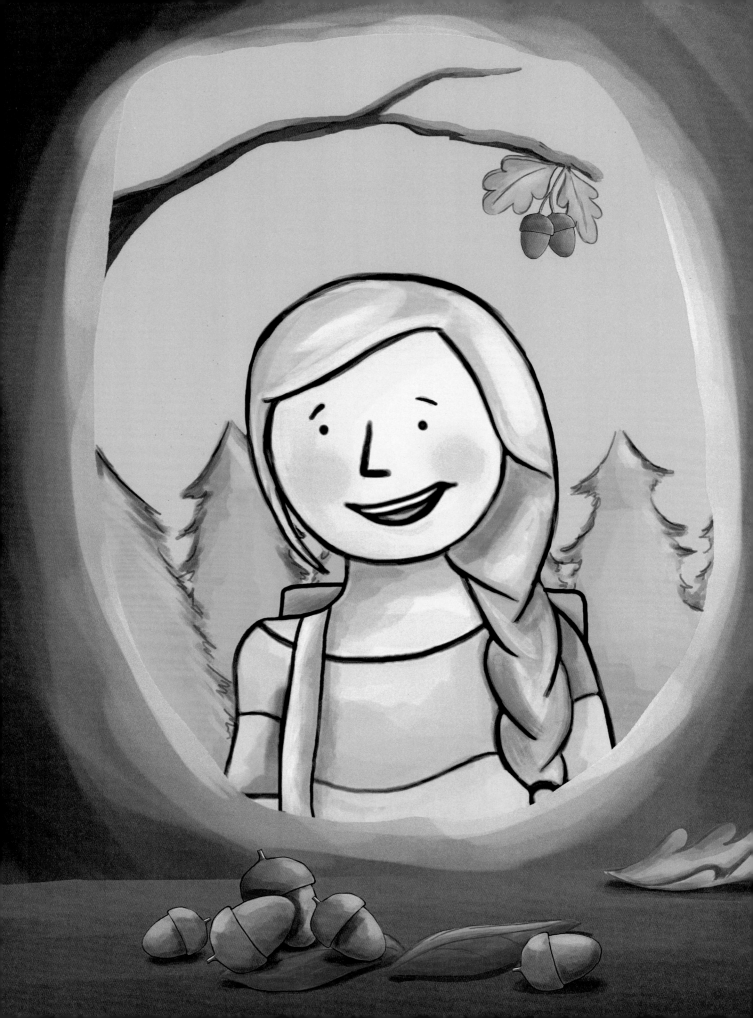

"Where do these nuts come from, Auntie Lisa?" Mia asked.

"From the trees!" Auntie Lisa shook a branch,
and acorns fell to the ground.
"Squirrels collect them for the winter."

Mia gathered a pile of acorns
and placed them into a tree hole.
"I wonder if squirrels get tired of eating acorns."

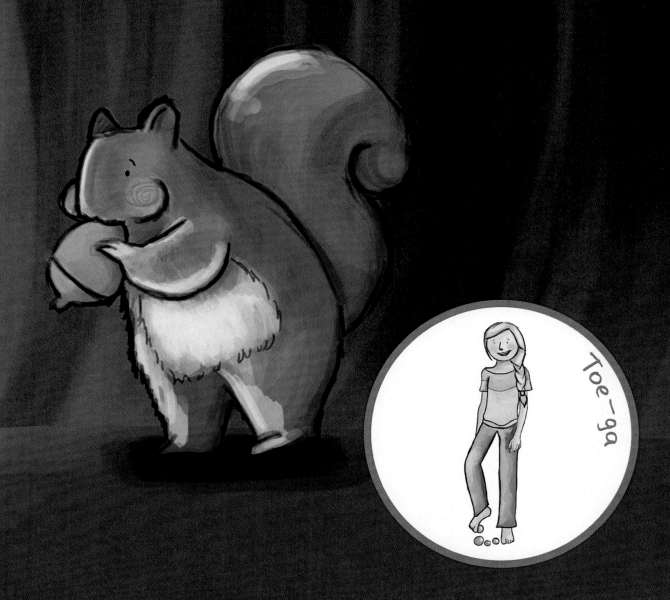

Toe—ga

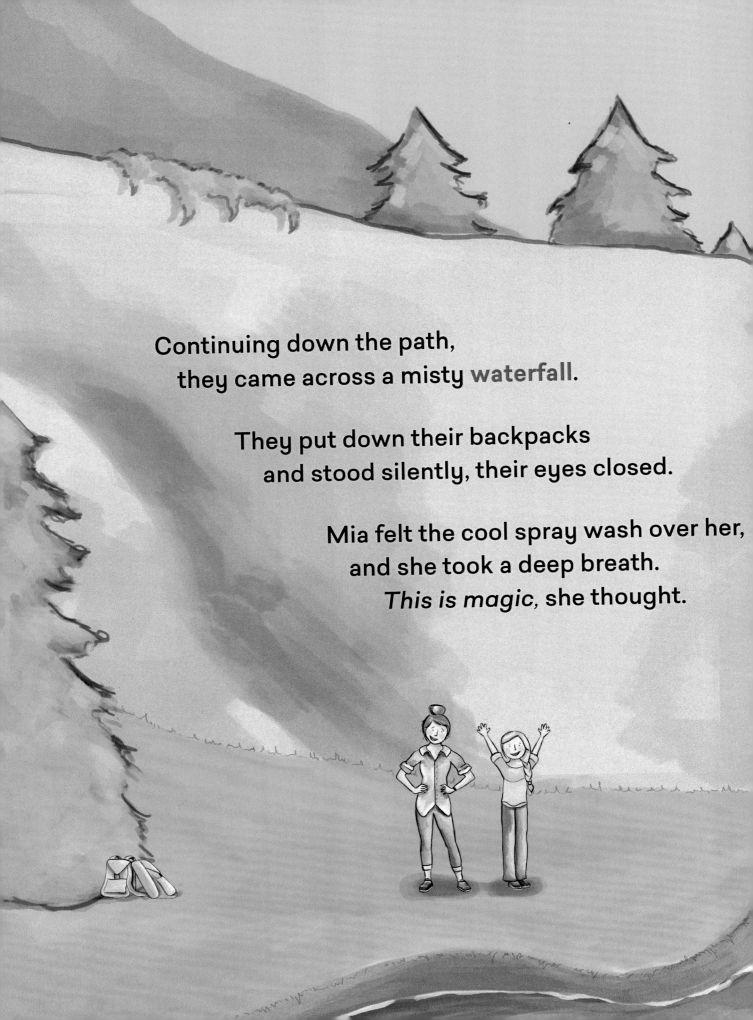

Continuing down the path,
they came across a misty **waterfall**.

They put down their backpacks
and stood silently, their eyes closed.

Mia felt the cool spray wash over her,
and she took a deep breath.
*This is magic*, she thought.

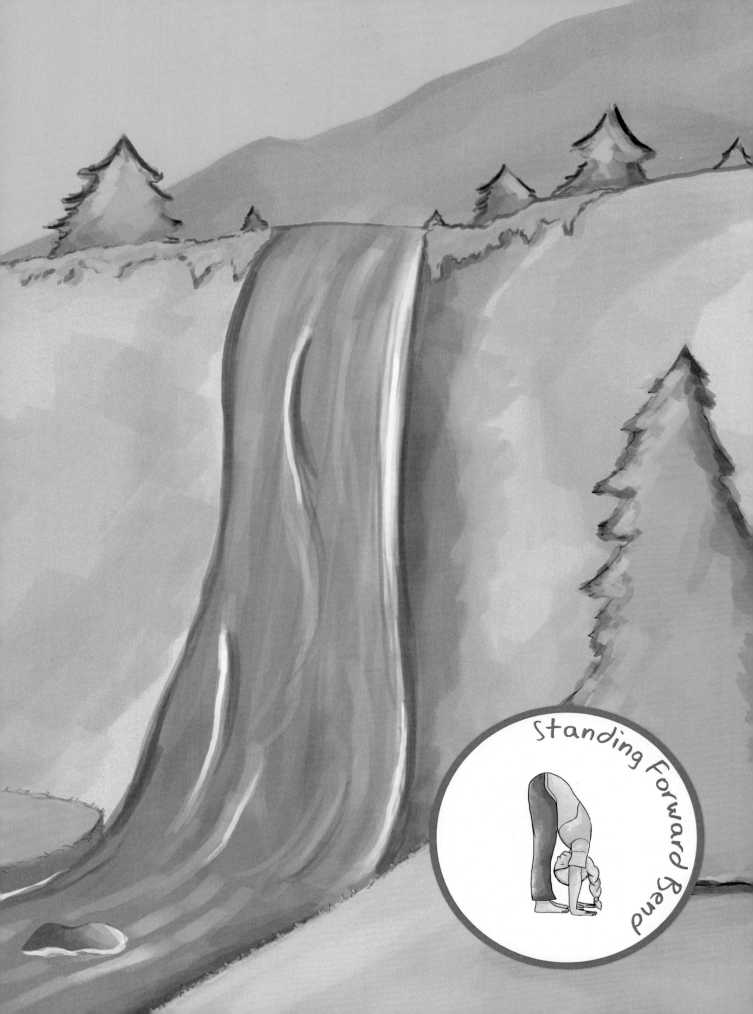

Standing Forward Bend

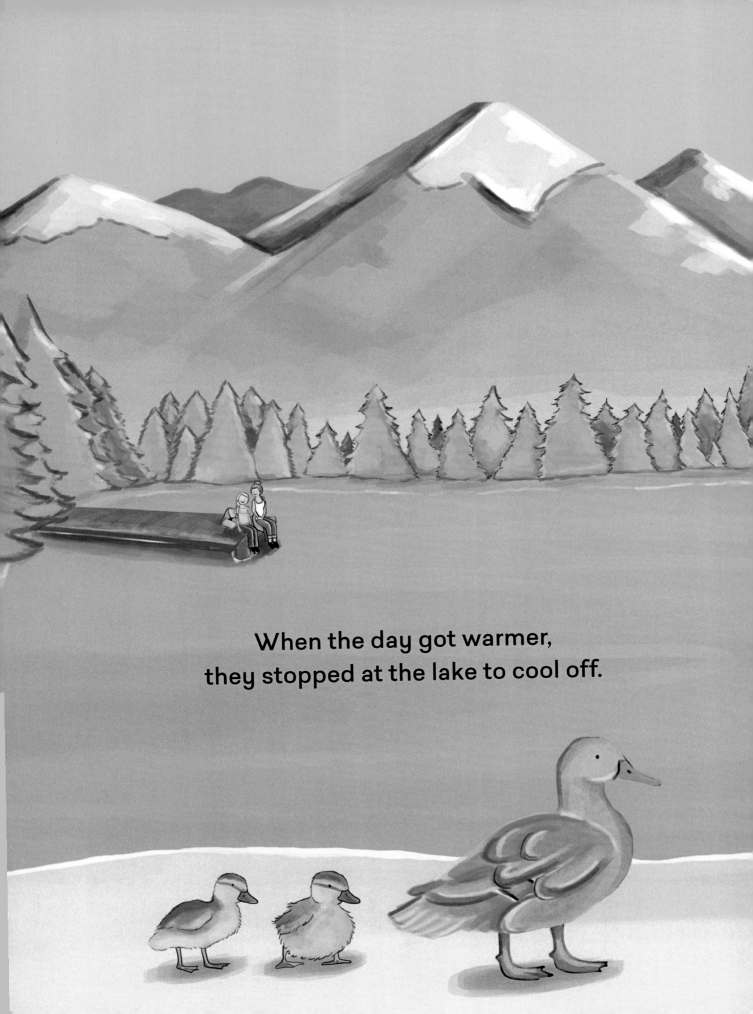

When the day got warmer,
they stopped at the lake to cool off.

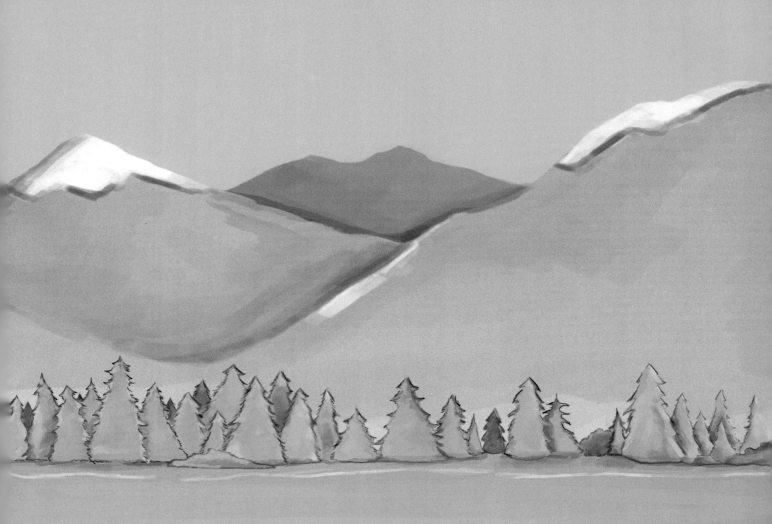

They watched a family of ducks
waddle past on the sandy beach.

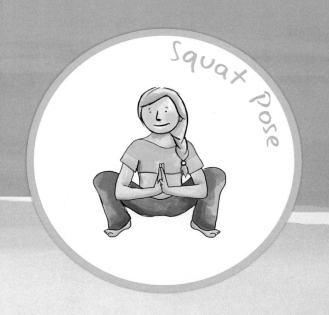

Squat Pose

Auntie Lisa pointed across the lake—
at a mama bear and her cubs.

"Stay still, Mia," she said, pulling Mia close.
"Those bears are busy eating berries
and aren't interested in us."

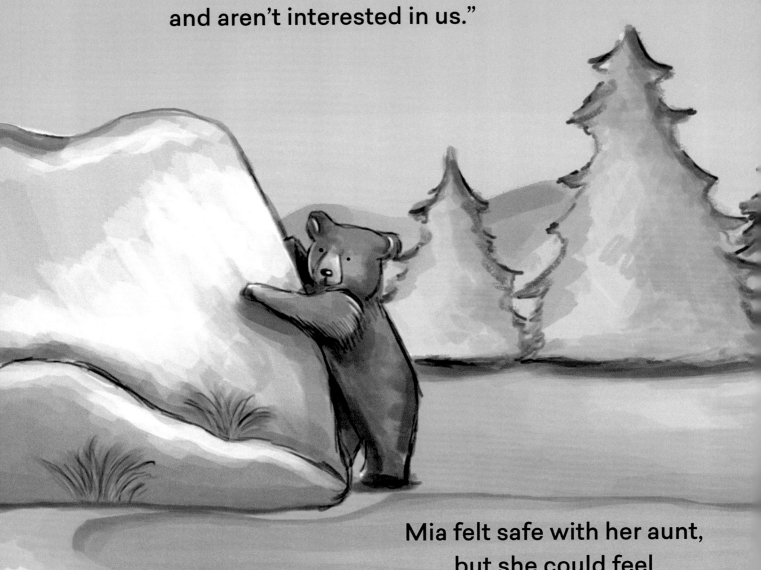

Mia felt safe with her aunt,
but she could feel
her heart beating faster.

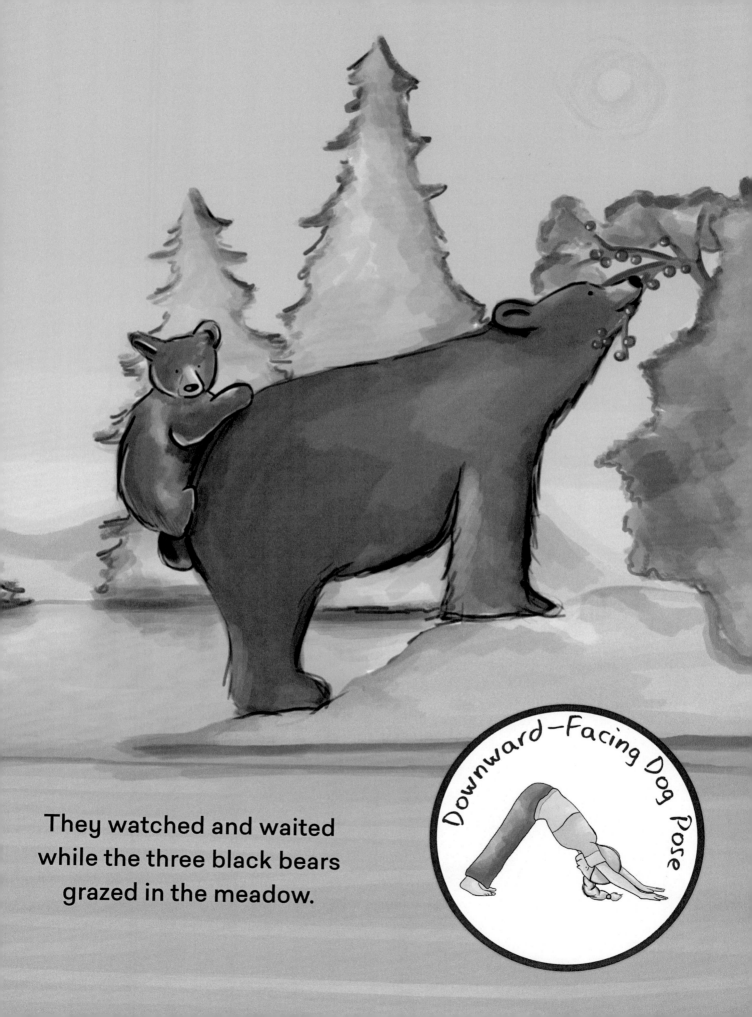

They watched and waited while the three black bears grazed in the meadow.

Downward-Facing Dog Pose

"Are bears dangerous, Auntie Lisa?"
Mia asked after the animals had ambled away.

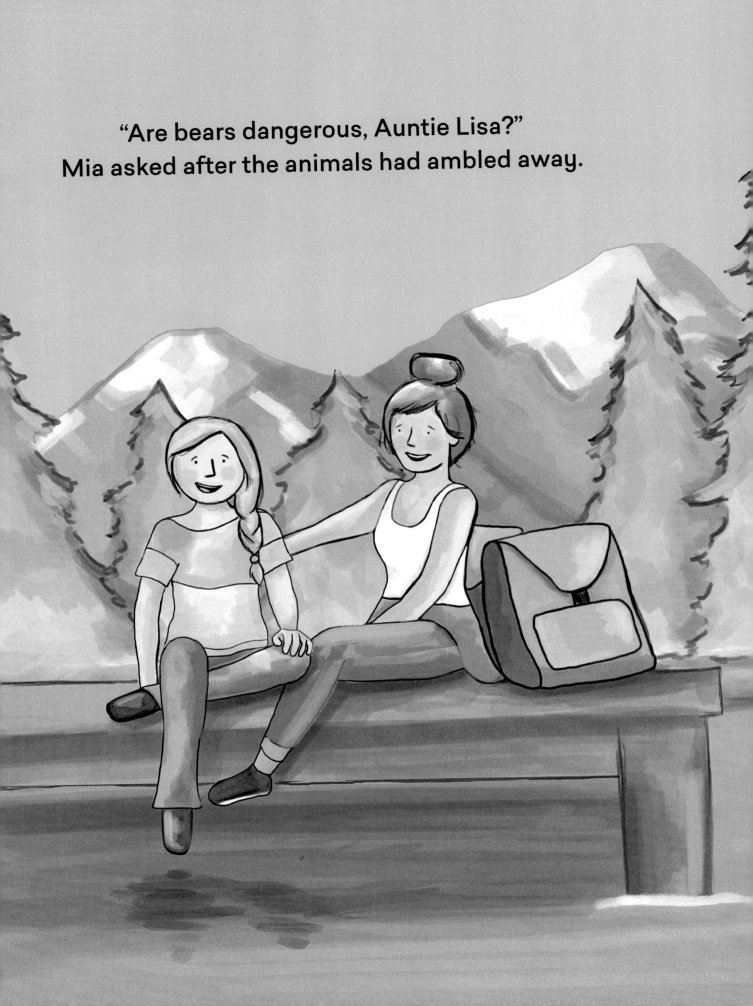

"That's a good question.
Bears aren't dangerous if we leave them alone.
The same goes for most wild animals."
Auntie Lisa patted her on the back.

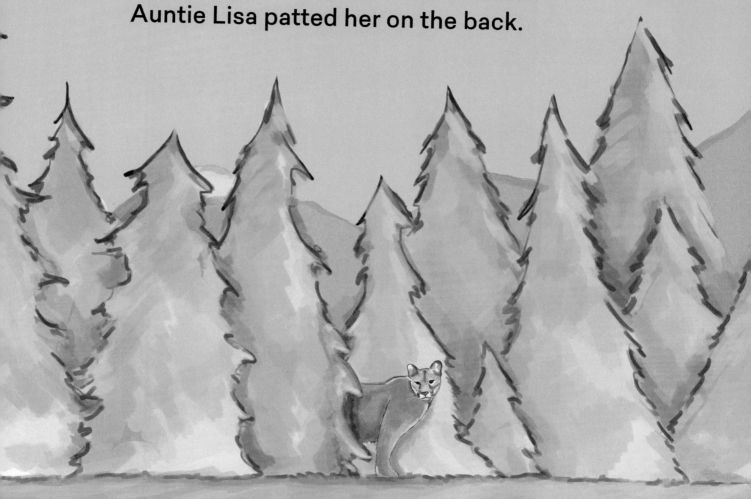

"Oh, like cougars?" asked Mia.

"Yes!" said her aunt.

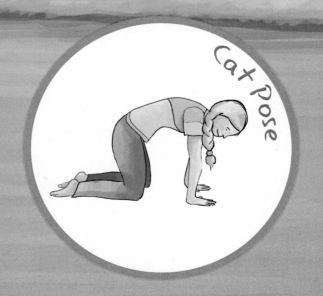

Cat Pose

Mia heard a rustle in the grass.
"I think I just heard a **snake**!"

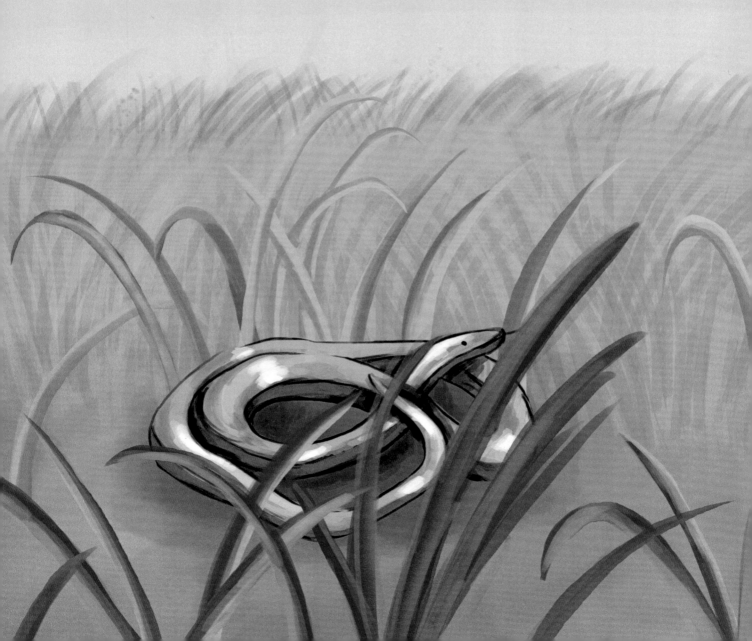

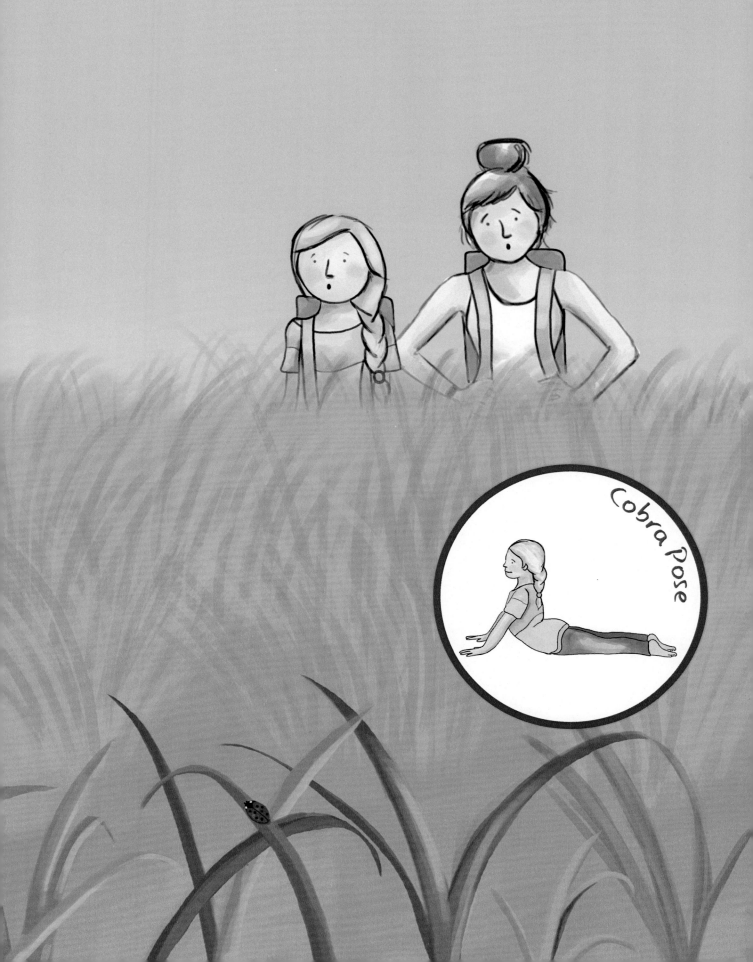

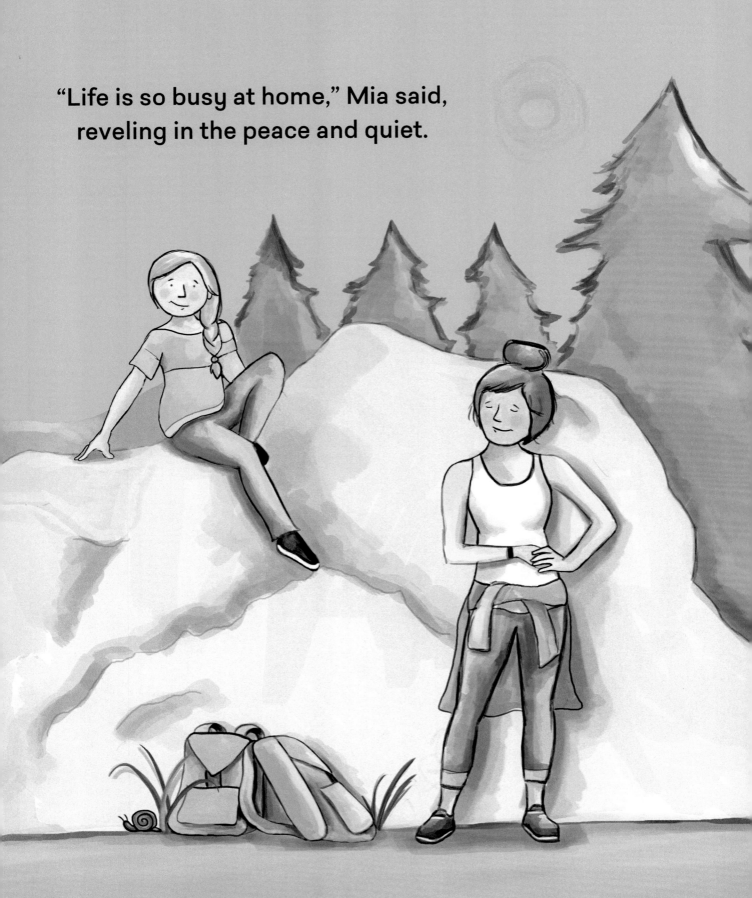

"Life is so busy at home," Mia said, reveling in the peace and quiet.

"That's why it's important
to take it easy once in a while."
Auntie Lisa leaned back against a rock.

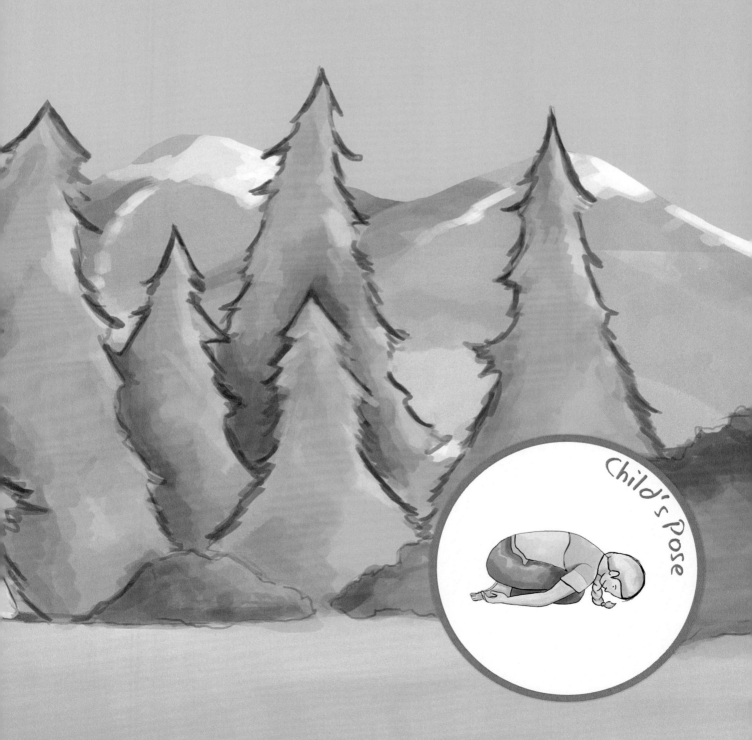

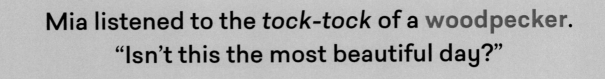

Mia listened to the *tock-tock* of a woodpecker.
"Isn't this the most beautiful day?"

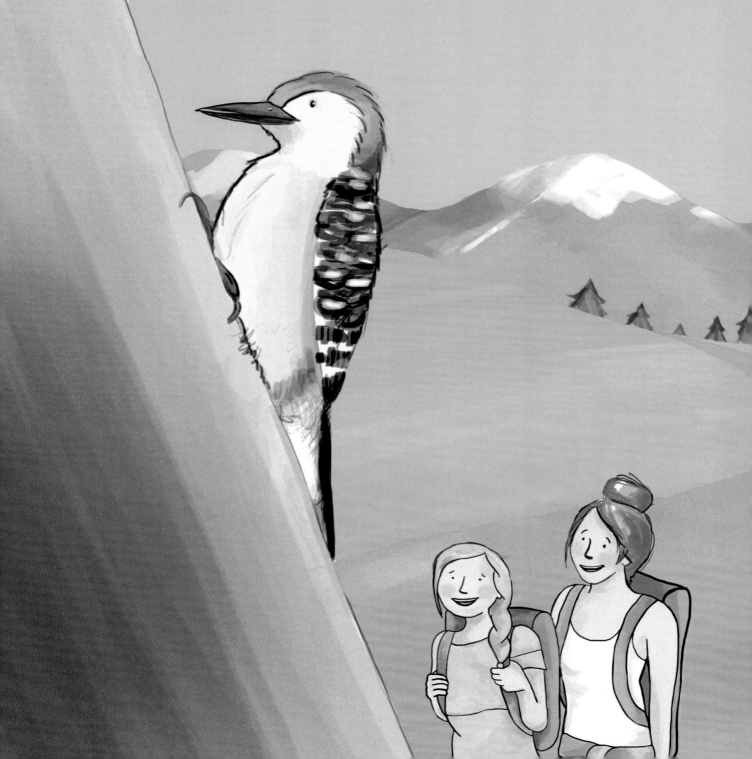

Auntie Lisa beamed.
"I think that woodpecker agrees with you!"

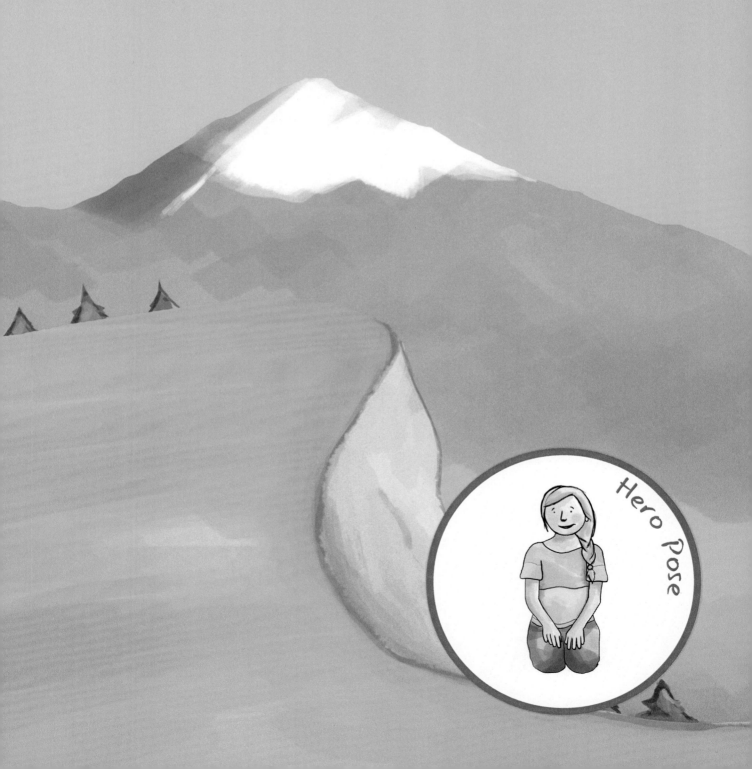

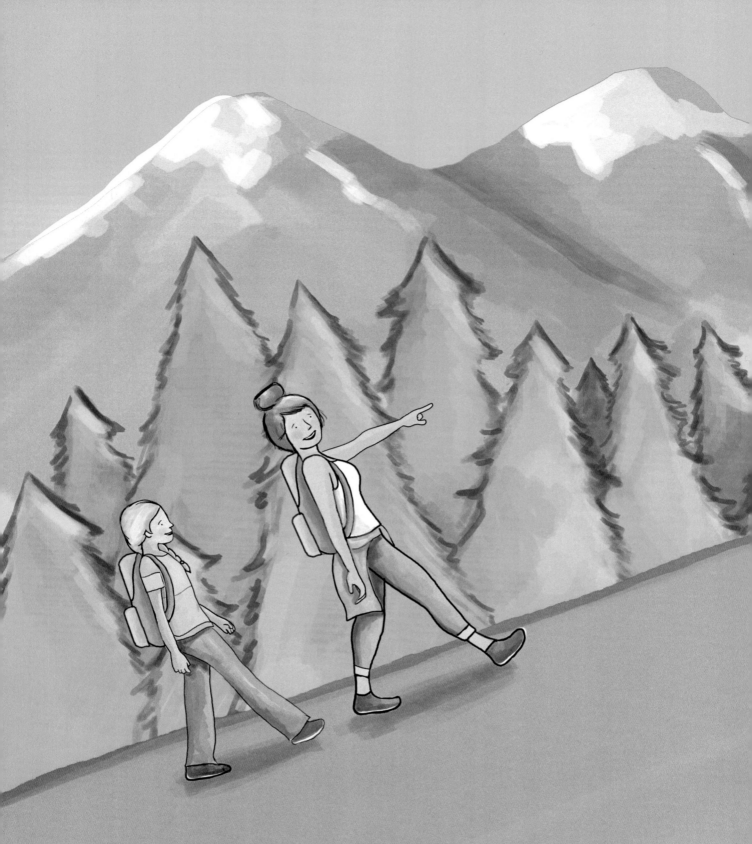

When they continued on their hike,
Auntie Lisa pointed out a deer
dashing up the hill beside them.

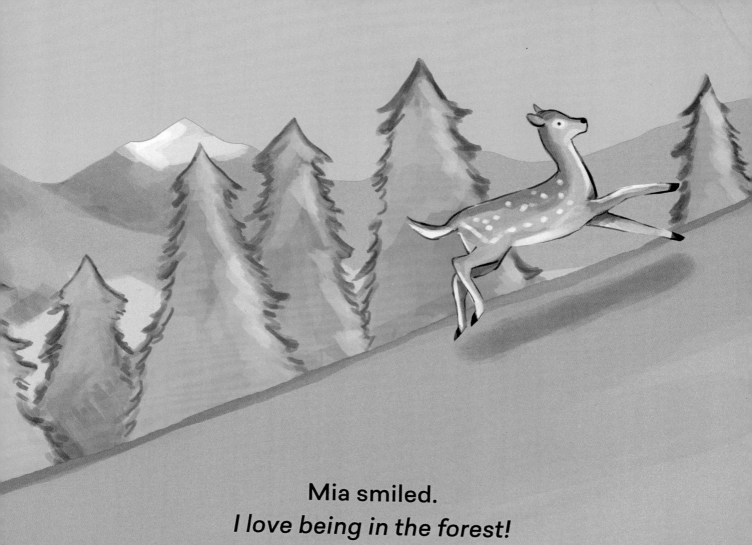

Mia smiled.
*I love being in the forest!*
she thought.

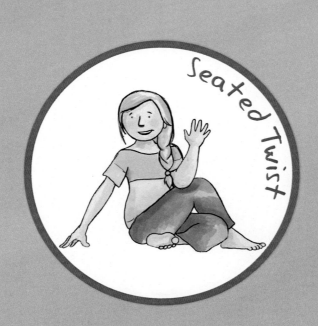

Seated Twist

Taking one step at a time,
they slowly climbed the rocky path.

Mia could hear her own **deep breathing**.

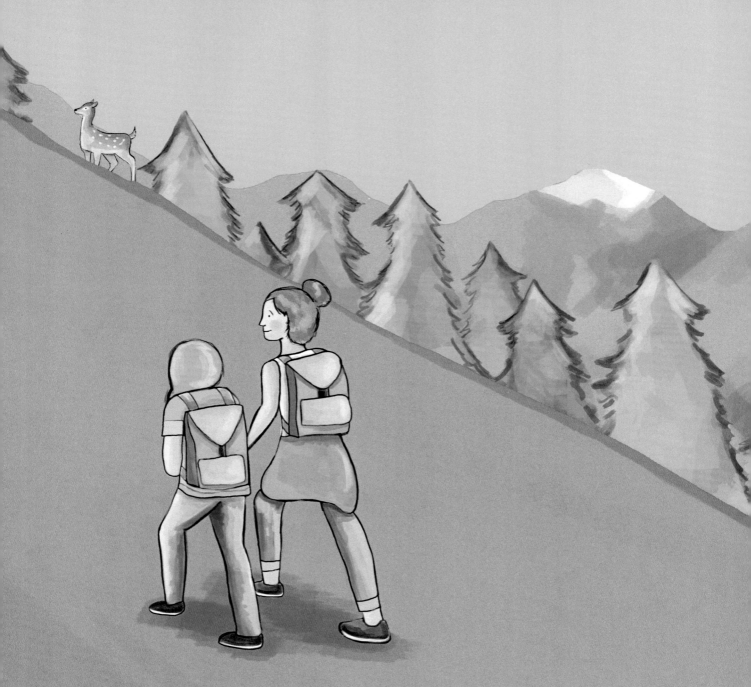

The deer had made the hike look easy,
but Mia had to focus and keep telling herself
that she could do it.

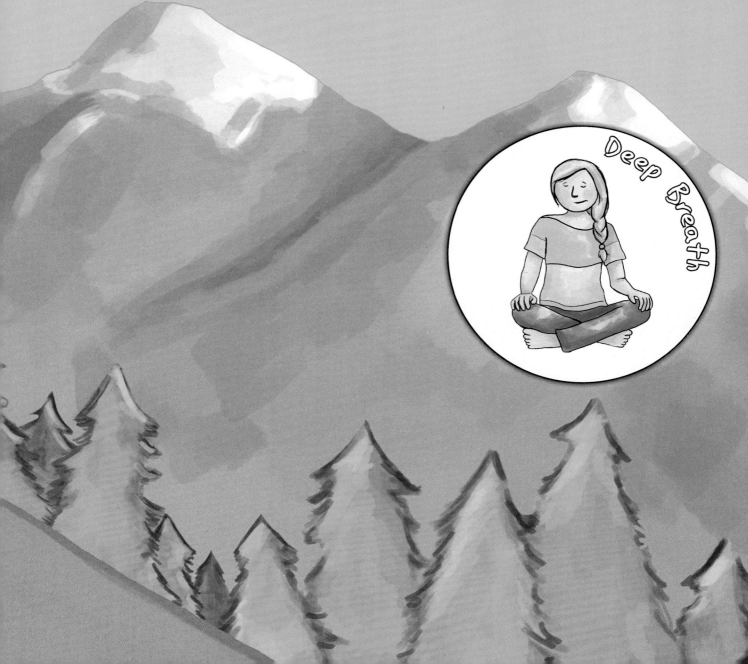

Finally, they came to a wooden bridge
crossing a rushing river.

"Where does the water come from, Auntie Lisa?"

"See how it comes down
from the top of the mountain?
Ice melts, and rain falls.
Then you have a river."

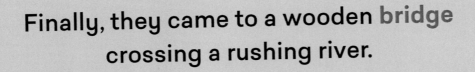

*There is so much to learn,* thought Mia.

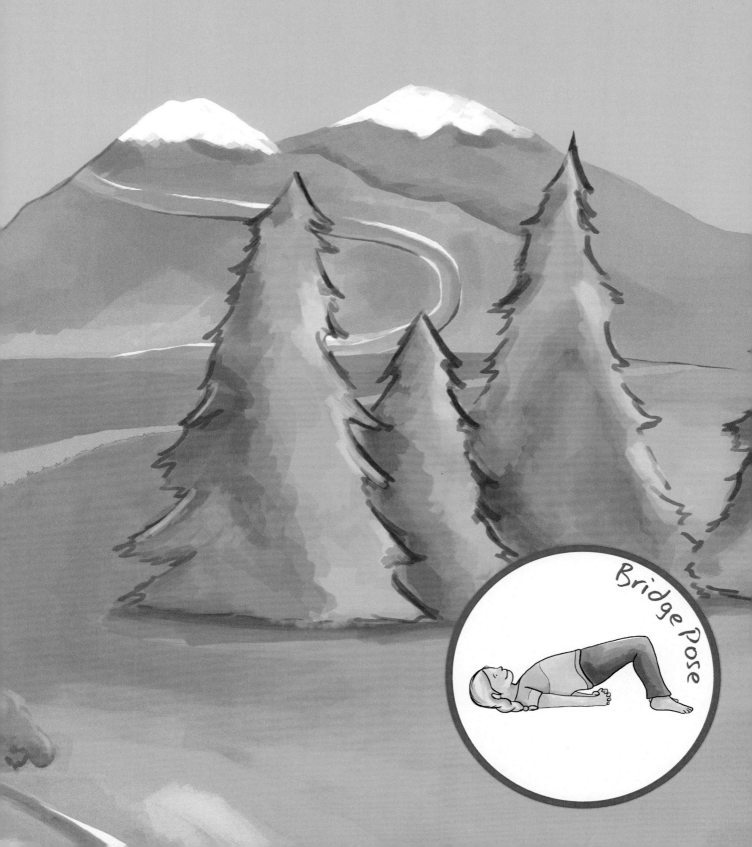

Bridge Pose

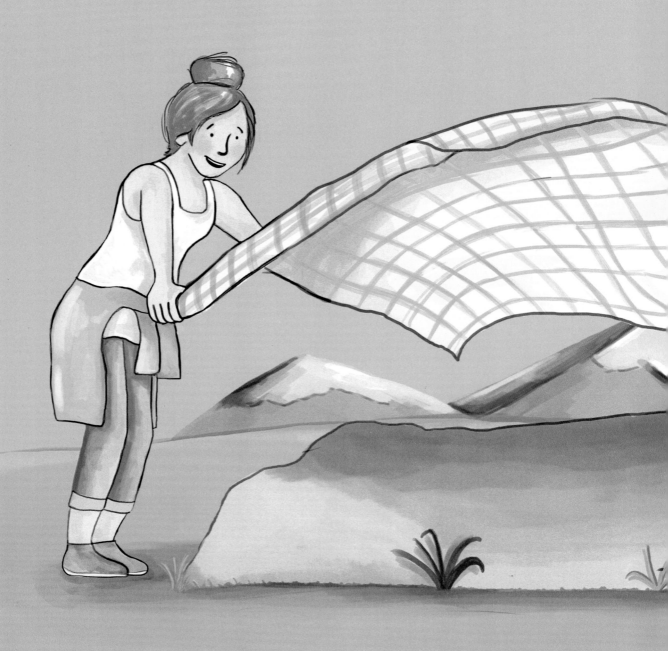

At the top of the mountain,
they used a flat rock as the **table** for their picnic.

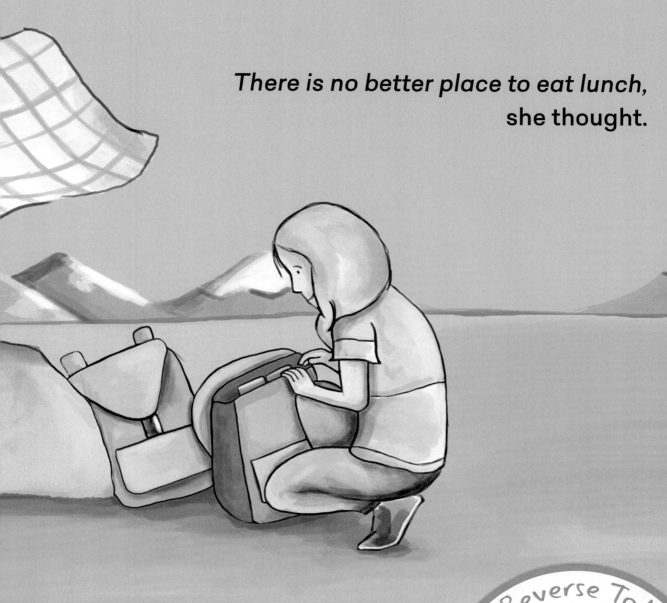

There is no better place to eat lunch,
she thought.

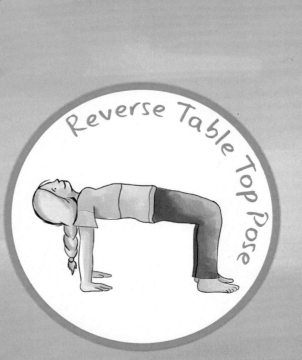

Reverse Table Top Pose

After lunch, they lingered at the summit.
Mia lay back and gazed at the blue sky.

The world seemed so big, and she felt so small.

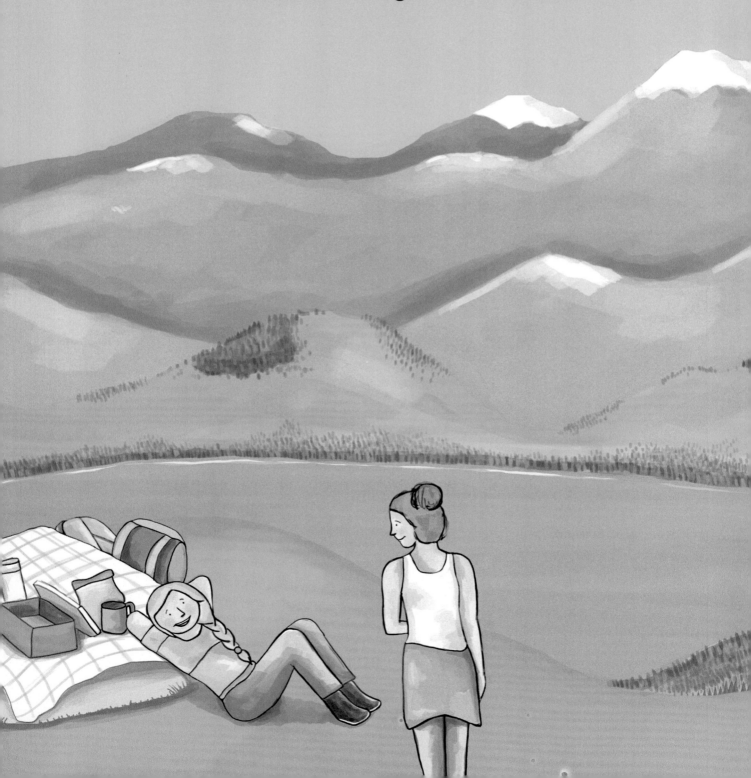

"Can we go on another hike soon?" Mia asked.

"You bet," said Auntie Lisa with a wink.

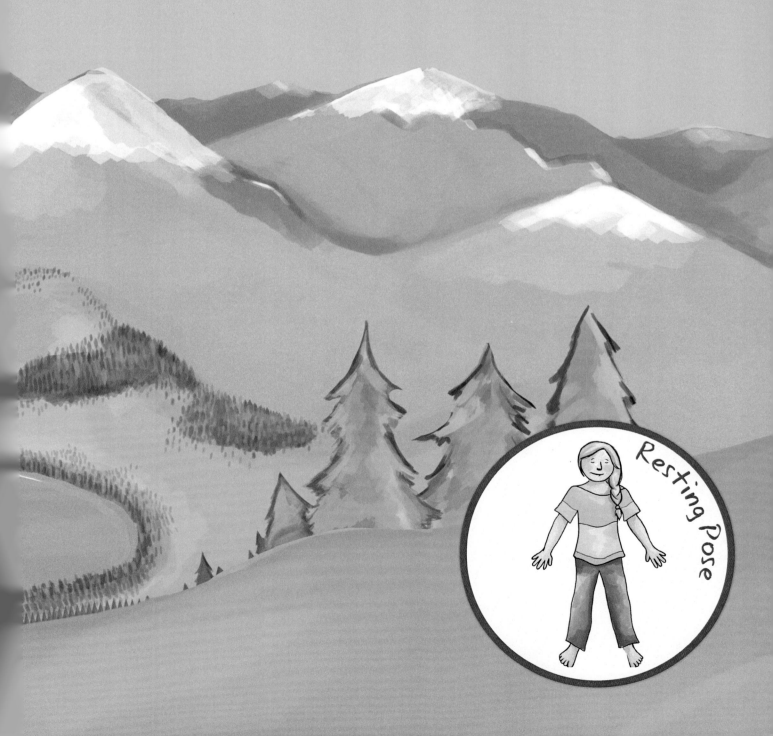

Resting Pose

# A Hike in the Forest

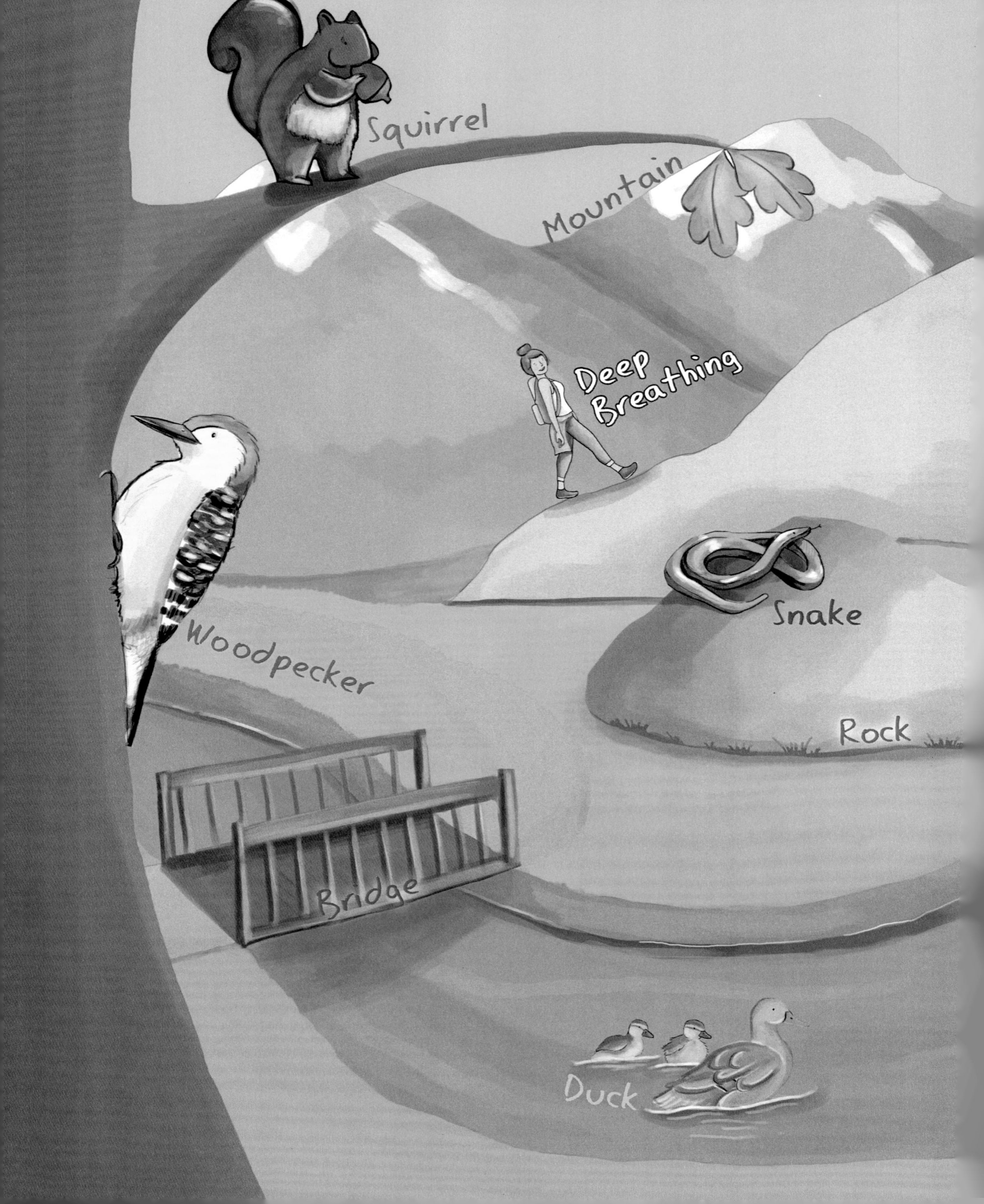

Squirrel

Mountain

Deep Breathing

Woodpecker

Snake

Rock

Bridge

Duck

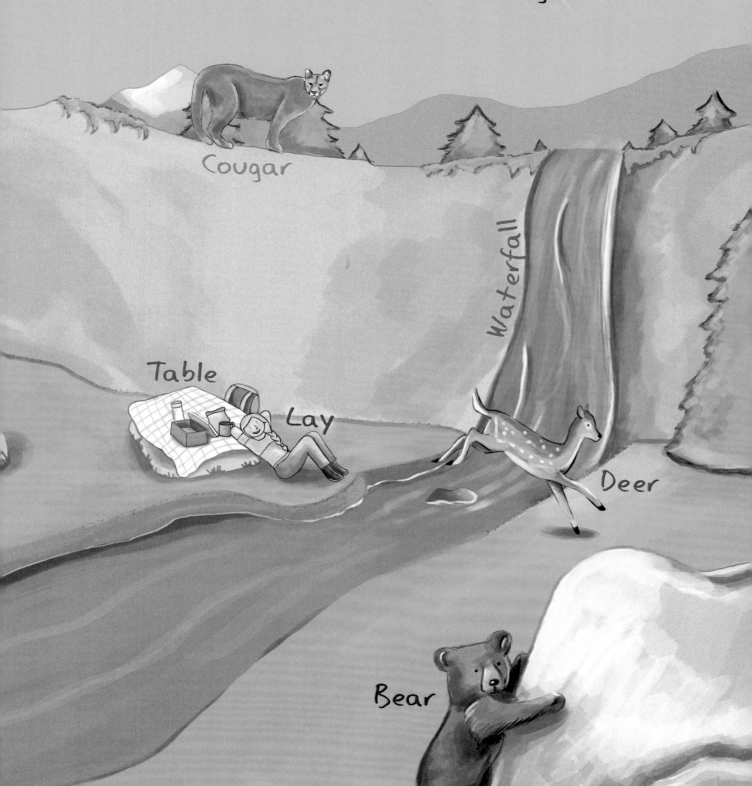

Eagle

Cougar

Table

Lay

Waterfall

Deer

Bear

# List of Yoga Poses for Kids

| # | Keyword | Yoga Pose | Demonstration |
|---|---------|-----------|---------------|
| 1. | Mountain | Mountain Pose | |
| 2. | Bald Eagle | Eagle Pose | |
| 3. | Squirrel | Toe-ga | |
| 4. | Waterfall | Standing Forward Bend | 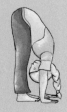 |
| 5. | Duck | Squat Pose | 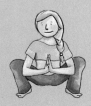 |

| # | Keyword | Yoga Pose | Demonstration |
|---|---------|-----------|---------------|
| 6. | Black Bear | Downward-Facing Dog Pose | |
| 7. | Cougar | Cat Pose | |
| 8. | Snake | Cobra Pose | |
| 9. | Rock | Child's Pose | |
| 10. | Woodpecker | Hero Pose | |

| # | Keyword | Yoga Pose | Demonstration |
|---|---------|-----------|---------------|
| 11. | Deer | Seated Twist | |
| 12. | Deep Breathing | Deep Breath | |
| 13. | Bridge | Bridge Pose | |
| 14. | Table | Reverse Table Top Pose | |
| 15. | Lay | Resting Pose | |

# How to Practice the Yoga Poses

The following list is intended as a guide only. Please encourage the children's creativity while ensuring their safety.

## Mountain Pose

Stand tall with your legs hip-width apart and feet facing forward. Take your arms straight alongside your body and imagine being a steady, tall mountain.

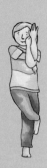

## Eagle Pose

Stand tall in Mountain Pose. Wrap your left leg around your right. Bring your bent arms out in front of you, wrap your right arm around your left arm, and bend your knees slightly. Pretend to perch in a tree like an eagle. Switch sides and repeat the steps.

## Toe-ga

Come back to standing tall. Put your hands on your hips. Now, lift one foot at a time, using your toes to pick up small, soft objects like pom-poms. Pretend to be squirrels collecting acorns in the forest.

## Standing Forward Bend

Stand tall with legs hip-width apart, feet facing forward, and straighten your arms alongside your body. Bend your upper body, reach for your toes, and pretend to be water falling over a waterfall.

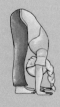

## Squat Pose

Come down to a squat with your arms bent like the wings of a duck. Waddle around like a duck on the sandy beach.

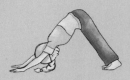

## Downward–Facing Dog Pose
Step back to your hands and feet in an upside-down V shape, with your buttocks up in the air, and pretend to be a bear eating berries.

## Cat Pose

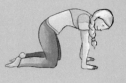

Press up and come to all fours on your hands and knees. Round your back and tuck your chin into your chest. Pretend to be a cougar hiding behind a tree.

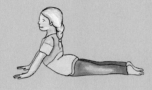

## Cobra Pose
Lie on your tummy and place your palms flat next to your shoulders. Pressing into your hands, lift your head and shoulders off ground. Hiss like a snake slithering in the grass.

## Child's Pose

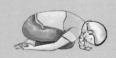

Sit on your heels, slowly bring your forehead down to rest on the floor in front of your knees, rest your arms down alongside your body, and take a few deep breaths. Pretend to be a rock beside the water's edge.

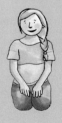

## Hero Pose
Come back to rest upright on your heels with your palms resting on your knees. Pretend to be a woodpecker pecking at a tree.

## Seated Twist

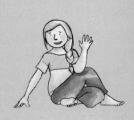

Start by sitting cross-legged, bend your right knee, and place your right foot behind your left knee. Check that your spine is straight and your right foot is flat on the ground. Twist your upper body to the right. Take your left elbow to your right knee and your right hand back behind you. Pretend to be a deer sitting in a meadow. Repeat on the other side.

## Deep Breath

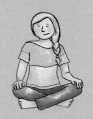

Come to sitting comfortably cross-legged, resting your palms on your knees. Close your eyes if that feels comfortable. Take a few deep breaths in and a few deep breaths out, relaxing your body.

## Bridge Pose

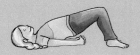

Lie on your back with your knees bent and your feet flat on the ground. Rest your arms down alongside your body, with your palms flat on the ground. Tuck your chin into your chest and keep your spine straight. On an inhale, lift your buttocks to imagine being a bridge across a rushing river.

## Reverse Table Top Pose

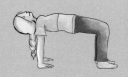

Come to sitting with your palms flat behind you and the soles of your feet flat in front of you. Lift your buttocks to create a long line from your head to your toes. Pretend to be a flat rock on the top of the mountain.

## Resting Pose

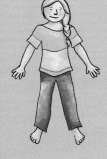

Lie on your back with your arms and legs stretched out. Breathe and rest. Imagine being on the mountain top smelling the fresh air and listening to the breeze.

# Parent-Teacher Guide

This guide contains tips to get the most out of your experience of yoga stories with young children.

**Put safety first.** Ensure that the space is clear and clean. Spend some time clearing any dangerous objects or unnecessary items. Wear comfortable clothing and practice barefoot.

**Props are welcome.** Yoga mats or towels (on a non-slip surface) are optional. Forest-related props and forest-themed music are good additions.

**Cater to the age group.** Use this Kids Yoga Stories book as a guide, but make adaptations according to the age of your children. Feel free to lengthen or shorten your journey to ensure that your children are fully engaged throughout your time together. We recommend reading this book with children ages three to six (preschoolers to early primary).

**Talk together.** Engage your children in the book's topic. Talk about what they know about the forest or their favorite forest books so they can form meaningful connections. Explain the purpose of yoga stories–to integrate movement, reading, and fun.

**Learn through movement.** Brain research shows that we learn best through physical activity. Our bodies are designed to be active. Encouraging your children to act out the keywords allows them to have fun while learning about forest life. Use repetition to engage the children and help them learn the movements. Ask your child to say or predict the next pose in their pretend forest hike.

**Develop breath awareness.** Throughout the practice, bring the children's attention to the action of inhaling and exhaling in a light-hearted way. For example, encourage the children to follow Mia as she takes a deep breath by the waterfall. Take time to breathe and relax in Child's Pose. Try a three-count inhale and a three-count exhale as she's climbing the rocky path.

**Relax.** Allow your children time to end their session in Resting Pose for five to ten minutes. Massage their feet during or after their relaxation period. Relaxation techniques give children a way to deal with stress. Reinforce the benefits and importance of quiet time for their minds and bodies. Introduce meditation, which can be as simple as sitting quietly for a couple of minutes, as a way to bring stillness to their highly stimulated lives.

**Lighten up and enjoy yourself.** A children's yoga experience is not as formal as an adult class. Encourage the children to use their creativity and provide them time to explore the postures. Avoid teaching perfectly aligned poses. The journey is intended to be joyful and fun. Your children feed off your passion and enthusiasm. So take the opportunity to energize yourself, as well. Read and act out the yoga book together as a way to connect with each other.

# About Kids Yoga Stories

We hope you enjoyed your Kids Yoga Stories experience.

Visit www.kidsyogastories.com to:

**Receive updates.** For yoga tips, updates, contest giveaways, articles, and activity ideas, sign up for our free **Kids Yoga Stories Newsletter.**

**Connect with us.** Please share with us about your yoga journey. Send pictures of yourself practicing the poses or reading the story. Describe your journey on our social media pages (Facebook, Pinterest, Google+, Instagram, and Twitter).

**Check out free stuff.** Read our articles on books, yoga, parenting, and travel. Download one of our kids yoga lesson plans or coloring pages.

**Read or write a review.** Read what others have to say about our yoga books for kids or post your own review on Amazon or on our website. We would love to hear how you enjoyed this yoga book.

Thank you for your support in spreading our message of integrating learning, movement, and fun.

Giselle

Kids Yoga Stories
www.kidsyogastories.com
giselle@kidsyogastories.com
www.pinterest.com/kidsyogastories
www.facebook.com/kidsyogastories
www.twitter.com/kidsyogastories
www.amazon.com/author/giselleshardlow
www.goodreads.com/giselleshardlow
www.instagram.com/kidsyogastories

## About the Author

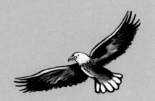

Giselle Shardlow draws from her experiences as a teacher, traveler, mother, and yogi to write her yoga stories for children. The purpose of her yoga books is to foster happy, healthy, and globally educated children. She lives in Boston with her husband and daughter.

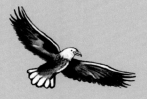

## About the Illustrator

Lauren Hughes resides in Gloucestershire, England. Her love for the outdoors and exploring nature can be seen throughout her work, with animals and flowers making frequent appearances. Her aim is to inspire and educate people through her drawings, to evoke emotions and to enhance understanding on many different levels.

# Other Yoga Books by Giselle Shardlow

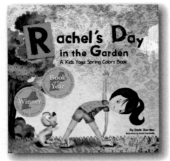

Rachel's Day
in the Garden

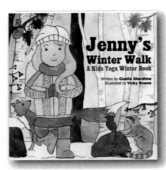

Jenny's Winter Walk

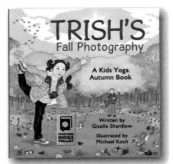

Trish's Fall Photography

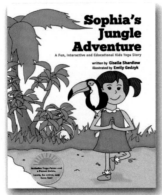

Sophia's Jungle
Adventure

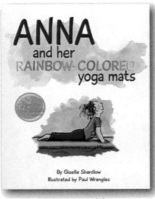

Anna and her
Rainbow-Colored
Yoga Mats

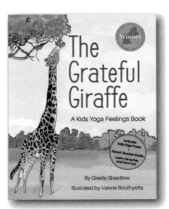

The Grateful Giraffe

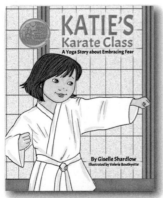

Katie's Karate Class

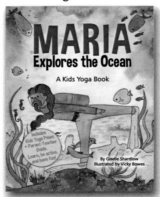

Maria Explores
the Ocean

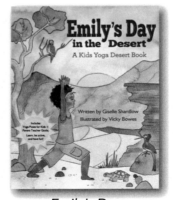

Emily's Day
in the Desert

Many of the yoga books above are available in multiple languages and eBook format.

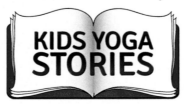

KIDS YOGA
STORIES

Buy your yoga books here: www.kidsyogastories.com

Made in the USA
San Bernardino, CA
17 March 2018